The Flexitarian Diet

How to lose weight, increase energy, and boost your immunity

Tim B. Rismo

i

ISBN: 9781710131789

Legal & Disclaimer

The information contained in this book and its contents is not designed to replace or take the place of any form of medical or professional advice; and is not meant to replace the need for independent medical, financial, legal or other professional advice or services, as may be required. The content and information in this book has been provided for educational and entertainment purposes only.

The content and information contained in this book has been compiled from sources deemed reliable, and it is accurate to the best of the Author's knowledge, information and belief. However, the Author cannot guarantee its accuracy and validity and cannot be held liable for any errors and/or omissions. Further, changes are periodically made to this book as and when needed. Where appropriate and/or necessary, you must consult a professional (including but not limited to your doctor, attorney, financial advisor or such other professional advisor) before using any of the suggested remedies, techniques, or information in this book.

Upon using the contents and information contained in this book, you agree to hold harmless the Author from and against any damages, costs, and expenses, including any legal fees potentially resulting from the application of any of the information provided by this book. This disclaimer applies to any loss, damages or injury caused by the use and application, whether directly or indirectly, of any advice or information presented, whether for breach of contract, tort, negligence, personal injury, criminal intent, or under any other cause of action.

You agree to accept all risks of using the information presented inside this book. You agree that by continuing to read this book, where appropriate and/or necessary, you shall consult a professional (including but not limited to your doctor, attorney, or financial advisor or such other advisor as needed) before using any of the suggested remedies, techniques, or information in this book.

TABLE OF CONTENT

INTRODUCTION

Flexible vegetarians or occasional carnivores are inclined to a healthy diet, flexible and without regrets. A sensible diet that seeks progress, not perfection.

Too often, diets are based on what you can't eat. You end up becoming too obsessed with eating a specific way that interferes with your lives. Perhaps this is why the flexitarian diet is a breath of fresh air in the world of diets.

Popular culture and foodies fill hashtags networks like #eatclean ("eat clean" in terms of sustainable, ecological, and healthy). According to Euromonitor International, meat is facing a decline in popularity in some European countries with a 15% reduction in consumption over the last decade. New vegetarian products have doubled in the last five years, providing better alternatives to meat. Perhaps we are only returning to a balance since, as many specialists say, we eat much more meat than we need. People become aware of how meat consumption affects climate change, our health, and our resources.

CHAPTER 1

WHAT IS A FLEXITARIAN DIET?

To know the origin of this term, we must first speak of millennials. They are young people born between 1980 and 1995, consumers born from technology, who love to eat and cook. The foodie generation. They lead the Social Networks in search of experiences and the tastiest gastronomy. It is said that they are the best trained in history and therefore the most demanding, who know what they want and do not conform. Food is one of its centers of interest along with social responsibility.

This social group has increased the consumption of unprocessed products in recent years, declaring themselves as devotees of healthy and sustainable products. They consume more outside the home and most of the time during the week. Celebrations and special occasions happen to be celebrated at home where they can cook for others. They can spend hundreds of euros on the latest technology or the latest fashion garments, but when eating out, they look for quality at a reduced price, even queuing up if the product is worth it. They are open to experimenting with any food, as citizens of the world they are, the more exotic and tasty the food, the greater the pleasure it will give them to try it. However, they are consumers in-store premises, with top quality products where they know first-hand the origin of what they are going to consume. They prefer to pay a little more for quality products.

Millennials seek the authenticity of things; they seek to feel different from the rest. They are not loyal customers, because they are constantly searching for new experiences and products, but they are grateful for the good treatment. They are responsible for the environment so that everything ecological and responsible for society will attract them. Millennials have a different food idea from the rest of the generations; they love to share a table at lunchtime, have dinner with strangers, and go shopping in a group. These young people seek a healthy lifestyle where good nutrition and sports are their main values.

With the arrival of this new and vindictive generation, different ways of consuming food have come to our society. We already know the followers of vegetarian and vegan diets, but... what about those in between? Are they one of those who ask for croquettes at home in Madrid?

What is flexitarianism?

This term was first used in 1992 by chef Helga Morath to define the menu of his new restaurant. It has reached our times by the foodies (food and beverage enthusiasts) as a healthy and balanced meal that does not force you to give up anything.

This diet consists of eating a diet based on fruits, vegetables, legumes, seeds, and cereals, combining it with meat intake sporadically and on time. These meats can be both beef and chicken and fish. Many will think that this diet is normal and current but in a balanced way, but no. The difference is that meat is only consumed at specific times and most, twice a week. When they consume mostly products at lower costs than meat, when they are going to buy it, they prefer to pay something more and consume high-quality products.

It is said to be a flexible diet derived from vegetarianism, but it is not so.

How is it different from vegetarianism?

Flexitarianism differs from vegetarianism in that the first one consumes dairy, eggs, and honey constantly, just like eating meat sporadically. If a vegetarian consumed meat, he would be breaking his strict diet, feeling remorse after it. Many consider it semi-vegetarianism, but as we have already said, with the intake of dairy, egg, and honey, it is no longer a derivative of vegetarianism.

The one that does go into semi-vegetarianism is ovolactovegetarianism that introduces eggs and dairy products into its diet without including meat. Many of the people who claim to be vegetarians are ovolácteovegetarianos because it is so complicated to carry out such a strict diet and consume foods that contain eggs and milk. As can be the croquettes, they eat boletus croquettes or candied leek, date, and carrot croquettes, but they cannot consume Iberian ham croquettes or cod croquettes.

In short, they can eat gourmet croquettes, but it depends on what they carry inside, they will be suitable for them or not.

Reasons to adopt a flexitarian diet

This trend is due to easy access to organic, organic and biological food. Every day there are more healthy proposals in the menus of the menu of the restaurants and many establishments that offer tasty and varied options.

Consciousness and food ethics also play a very important role in this fashion that does not seem temporary. The millennials are very sensitive to show the animal welfare or the great cost of the consumption of meat to the environment from CO2 emissions to the growing need for space for growing food for animals (that results in, for example, deforestation of the Amazon rainforest). The resources used are exorbitant: approximately 16,000 liters of water are needed to produce a kilo of veal.

Recently, many documentaries showing animal cruelty and the risks of eating meat for the environment and health have been issued. Red meat is high in fat, salt, and chemicals related to cardiovascular disease and cancer. In addition, the excessive use of antibiotics in intensive industrial farms contributes to greater resistance to antibiotics in humans.

Many opt for better quality meat: poultry, grass-fed beef, wild fish. On the other hand, they avoid processed meats such as salami, sausages, bacon. The economic aspect is also very important. The reduction in meat and fish intake means that families spend less in general on their food and meat budgets of inferior quality.

CHAPTER 2

THE BENEFITS OF THE
FLEXITARIAN DIET

The food flow based on the balance of food that gains strength.

If there is something that cannot be denied, it is that food is fashionable. Foodies trends are always being renewed, and there is an incredible offer of diet possibilities that allows each one to choose the one that best suits their personality or needs.

Among the different options, there is a food flow that is presented as the healthiest or most balanced: flexitarianism. It is based on promoting the intake of fruits, vegetables, and legumes and rationing the consumption of meat or fish.

In other words, a vegetarian diet that is complemented with some products of animal origin, such as fish, shellfish, poultry, or meat, although they do not have to be all; Some people choose only a few of them.

However, although the term flexitarianism is a mixture of the word vegetarian and flexible, people who follow this type of food are not vegetarians because they consume products of animal origin automatically excluded from this group.

For these people, eating meat or fish does not imply a violation of their ideals or diet model. Some initiatives take this concept of flexitarianism and are inspired by it for certain customs. Examples of them are the Meat Free Mondays, which drives among other celebrities Paul Mccartney or Vegan Before 6 (Vegan before six) emerged from the imagination of The New York Times culinary critic Mark Bittman.

Benefits

Experts agree that it is a healthy diet because it combines the benefits of products of plant origin with the nutrients provided by sporadic intake of those of animal origin. One of the main recommendations of nutritionists and doctors to maintain good health through food is to consume at least five pieces of fruit and vegetables a day and reduce the intake of processed foods.

That is why this food option is qualified as healthy. It is low in saturated fat and cholesterol and high in nutrients and fiber and protects cardiovascular health. To these advantages are added the punctual contributions of Omega 3 fatty acids found in fish and high-quality proteins and vitamin B12 that come from meats.

The flexitarian diet can have many benefits for the human being since it is an extremely healthy diet, which is very similar to the vegetarian with the option of eating meat and fish in small quantities. You will lose weight and get a healthier lifestyle.

It gives you more life

Eating too much meat shortens life. But with the flexitarian diet, you can live three and a half years more according to a study. This is due to the amount of fiber, good carbohydrates and antioxidants than foods consumed throughout the day have.

Less disease

All health experts prove junk food sick and. Many people have a higher risk of suffering from cancer and cardiovascular diseases because they lead to this lifestyle. But with the flexitarian diet, fruits, vegetables, and grains will greatly improve your health, and you will feel better than ever.

You lose weight

By eating so healthy it is obvious that you will be able to lose weight healthily, vegetarians also do it, but they have less body mass than they should, but as in this regime you eat meat, lose weight and your body mass is adequate.

Aid for the environment

It is one of the main reasons why people join vegetarianism since they take care of animals and avoid damaging the environment with many products used in hatcheries. Growing plants is very good for the land, so by doing so, you have the option that you can grow more and more.

Meat and fish of good quality

Ideally, you get meat and fish of very good quality, that is, those that are lean protein, with the lowest possible fat content. Vegetables are cheaper, so you will not mind spending a little more on the small portions of meat and fish that you will eat per month to be of the best kinds.

A flexitarian diet would reduce the chances of being obese by half, according to a recent study carried out by several experts from the University of Navarra. The research used a sample of 16,000 university graduates, whose eating habits and evolution were analyzed from 1999 and for a decade.

CHAPTER 3

FLEXITARIAN DIET: TWO WEEKS OF MENUS

Eat less meat and more plant: this is the new winning equation to lighten up a few pounds. It's not that hard to prepare good, balanced, light meals with little animal protein! Just follow our flexitarian menus...

Aurélia Huchet, the dietician, developed these menus that showcase plants. They respect the key principles of flexitarianism, a new food practice, both healthy and destocking.

Week 1 of flexitarians menus

Monday

<table>
<tr><td>

Breakfast

- Cinnamon infusion, ginger, lemon
- One kiwi
- One egg
- Two slices of wholemeal bread (50 g)

</td><td>

Lunch

- Endive salad and walnuts (20 g), vinaigrette (1 tbsp walnut oil)
- 150 g of quinoa
- Pan-parsnip (1 tbsp olive oil)
- 100 g pistachio pudding

</td></tr>
</table>

Dinner

- Cream of butternut soup with turmeric
- Vegetable stew with kombu seaweed
- Three litchis

Kombu Algae Vegetable Stew Recipe

1. Preparation 15 min, cooking 40 min

2. For four pers. 6 to 8 sheets of Kombu seaweed, 800 g to 1 kg vegetable julienne, soy sauce, one onion, one garlic clove, pepper, herbs, olive oil

3. Soften the algae in water for 10 minutes. Keep the water. Cut them into thin slices and cook them with the vegetable julienne in the soaking water for 10 to 15 minutes.

4. In a skillet, fry the chopped onion in 1 tbsp. To s. Olive oil and some seaweed water. Add to the seaweed with a little soy sauce, chopped garlic, pepper, and herbs. Let simmer for 15 minutes.

Tuesday

Breakfast

- Two prunes
- Four c. to s. oatmeal
- 200 ml of almond milk
- 20 g of almonds

Lunch

- Grated carrots vinaigrette (1 tsp of rapeseed oil)
- Brunoise of sauteed vegetables with 100 g of tofu (1 tsp of olive oil)
- 100 g of mango compote

Dinner

- Onion soup and dulse
- One buckwheat pancake with mushrooms (1 tsp of olive oil)
- 100 g of cottage cheese (cow or goat)

Wednesday

Breakfast

- Green tea
- ½ banana
- Four wasa fibers
- One plain soy yogurt

Lunch

- Arugula salad with pumpkin seeds (20 g) vinaigrette (1 tbsp walnut oil)
- Coral lentils with seasonal vegetables
- 100 g of vegetable juice and vanilla rice

Dinner

- Pumpkin soup with curry
- 120 g of pollack with herbs (1 tsp of olive oil)
- Steamed broccoli
- One apple cooked with cinnamon

Thursday

Breakfast

- Star anise infusion
- Two clementines
- Two slices of spelled bread (50 g)
- 10 g of almond puree
- One sheep milk yogurt

Lunch

- Salad of mesclun with cashew nuts (20 g) vinaigrette (1 tsp of rapeseed oil)
- Stuffed cabbage with 100 g tofu
- 30 g of goat cheese

Dinner

- Root vegetable soup
- 150 g of rice with saffron and gourmet peas
- Parsley green beans (1 tbsp olive oil)
- One pear

Friday

Breakfast

- Cinnamon porridge (200 ml milk with 30 g oat flakes and cinnamon)
- Ten raisins
- Green tea

Lunch

- Apple carrot ginger juice
- Two egg omelets with chives (1 tablespoon olive oil)
- spinach
- 150 g of citrus salad

Dinner

- Mixed dry bean soup
- 100 g spaghetti of small spelled
- Fondue of leeks (1 tsp of olive oil)
- One plain soy yogurt

Saturday

Breakfast

- Green tea
- Two slices of sourdough bread (50 g)
- 10 g sesame puree
- One yogurt of cow or plain soy

Lunch

- Green salad with lemon juice
- Chinese chicken
- 150 g of fruit salad

Dinner

- Miso soup
- Steamed carrots with cumin and freshly roasted chestnuts (150 g)
- 100 g of vegetal dessert with coffee

Chinese chicken recipe

1. Preparation 10 min, cooking 25 min, waiting for two h

2. For six pers. 800 g of chicken breast, one red pepper, one green pepper, 150 g of onion, 150 g of celery, 200 g of black mushrooms, 150 g of bean sprouts, some spinach leaves, 2 tbsp. To s. Lime juice, 3 tbsp. to s. of olive oil, one chicken broth, salt and pepper

3. Marinate 1 to 2 hours in the fresh diced chicken with lemon juice and zest, oil, salt, and pepper. Brown in a nonstick skillet, add the minced vegetables (except spinach) and cook for 15-20 minutes. Add the spinach at the end.

4. Serve in a tureen with hot chicken broth.

Sunday

Breakfast

- Basswood infusion
- One blood orange
- Four c. to s. of muesli without added sugar
- 200 ml of goat's milk

Lunch

- Green salad with hazelnut chips (20 g) vinaigrette (1 teaspoon hazelnut oil)
- 120 g roasted king of seabream
- Fennel fondue (1 tablespoon of olive oil)
- 100 g of apple mushroom with verbena

Dinner

- Green vegetable soup
- 100 g of polenta
- Braised endive (1 tbsp olive oil)
- 30 g of sheep's cheese

Week 2 of flexitarians menus

Monday

Breakfast

- 150 ml of pomegranate juice
- 100 g of cottage cheese
- Two slices of spelled bread (50 g)
- 10 g of hazelnut puree
- Infusion with red vine

Lunch

- Mesclun with flax seeds (20 g) vinaigrette (1 tsp of rapeseed oil)
- 150 g of bulgur and mint beans
- Pan-fried vegetables (Jerusalem artichokes, parsnip) (1 tablespoon olive oil)
- One plain soy yogurt

Dinner

- Cream of leeks and rutabaga
- Pan-fried chard ribs, Chinese cabbage, and seaweed tempeh
- 100 g passion fruit compote

Recipe for fried chard ribs, Chinese cabbage, and seaweed tempeh

1. Preparation 10 min, baking 15 min

2. For four pers. 200 g of seaweed tempeh or 200 g of tempeh + 4 tsp. To s. of seaweed in flakes, eight ribs of cut-away chard, one shallot, one clove of garlic, 1 Chinese cabbage, 1 tbsp. To s. Soy sauce, 1 tbsp. To s. Vinegar, 1 tsp. To c. red sugar, oil

3. In a wok, fry the minced shallot in 1 tbsp. To c. Oil. When it begins to become translucent, add minced garlic, sugar, vinegar. Stir 1 min., Pour tempeh into cubes and add 1 to 2 tbsp. To s. of water. Cover and cook for 5 minutes. Add the vegetables. Cover and cook over medium heat, occasionally stirring until chard ribs are cooked but crisp. Season with soy sauce.

Tuesday

<table>
<tr><td>

Breakfast

- One kiwi
- Two slices of wholemeal bread (50 g)
- One eggshell
- Green tea

</td><td>

Lunch

- Cheese with hazelnut chips (20 g) vinaigrette (1 tbsp walnut oil)
- 120 g steamed vinaigrette with capers and diced lemon (1 tsp olive oil)
- Fallen spinach
- One apple

</td></tr>
</table>

Dinner

- Red bean soup with ginger
- Wheat tagliatelle duo (100 g) and carrots
- One natural yogurt of goat or cow

Wednesday

<table>
<tr><td>

Breakfast

- ½ banana
- Porridge with almond juice (200 ml + 30 g oat flakes)
- Star anise infusion

</td><td>

Lunch

- Salad of Oak Leaves Vinaigrette (1 tsp of rapeseed oil)
- 120 g of chicken breast with tarragon
- Salsify (1 teaspoon olive oil)
- Two tangerines

</td></tr>
</table>

Dinner

- Cream of azuki with laurel
- Millet gratin with broccoli
- One oat yogurt

Recipe of millet gratin with broccoli

1. Preparation 10 min, cooking 40 min

2. For four pers. 160 g millet semolina, 400 ml rice juice, two eggs, 600 g broccoli, salt, nutmeg, one clove of garlic

3. Wash the millet semolina and cook it in the salted rice juice (15 min on low heat, after boiling).

4. Steam broccoli and mix. Beat the eggs and add the nutmeg. Mix everything. Rub a garlic gratin dish and oil it. Put the mixture in a hot oven (Th.5) for about 15 min.

Thursday

Breakfast

- Star anise infusion
- Two clementines
- Two slices of spelled bread (50 g)
- 10 g of almond puree
- One sheep milk yogurt

Lunch

- Salad of mesclun with cashew nuts (20 g) vinaigrette (1 tsp of rapeseed oil)
- Stuffed cabbage with 100 g tofu
- 30 g of goat cheese

Dinner

- Root vegetable soup
- 150 g of rice with saffron and gourmet peas
- Parsley green beans (1 tbsp olive oil)
- One pear

Thursday

Breakfast

- Four c. to s. of muesli without added sugar to the dried fruits
- 200 ml of rice juice

Lunch

- Roquette with sesame seeds (20 g) vinaigrette (1 tbsp walnut oil)
- Pan-fried mushrooms and 100 g tofu (1 tsp olive oil)
- Two clementines

Dinner

- Celery soup with nutmeg
- 100 g green lentils with carrots and onions (1 tsp olive oil)
- 100g of tapioca with vegetable juice

Friday

Breakfast

- ½ grapefruit
- Two slices of sourdough bread (50 g)
- 10 g of almond puree
- One soy yogurt
- Green tea

Lunch

- Beet / apple / ginger juice
- Fennel crumble way
- One natural yogurt

Dinner

- Turnip soup with curry
- Two eggs with an herbed omelet (1 tsp of olive oil)
- Green salad with pine nuts (20 g) vinaigrette (1 tsp of rapeseed oil)
- 150 g of pineapple carpaccio

Recipe of fennel crumble the way

1. Preparation 15 min, cooking 30 min

2. For six pers. 4 to 6 fennel bulbs, 1 tbsp. to c. of olive oil, 1 tbsp. to c. of cumin, salt, and pepper. For the dough: 60 g rice flakes, 60 g rice flour, 1 tbsp. to s. flax seeds, salt

3. Chop the fennel. Sauté for 3 minutes with cumin and oil. Reduce heat, cover, and continue cooking for 15 minutes. Add ½ glass of water. Preheat the oven to 180 ° C. Prepare the crumble: in a bowl, wet the rice flakes with 1 tbsp. to s. Olive oil. Mix, add flour, and flaxseed. Salt and stir in water until the grains are tender. In a gratin dish, pour the fennel and cover with dough. Cook for 10 minutes in the oven.

Saturday

Breakfast

- One orange
- Four c. to s. rye flakes
- 200 ml of rice juice
- 20 g of almonds
- Rosemary infusion

Lunch

- Sprouted Scarole with Sprouted Seeds (1 tsp of rapeseed oil)
- 150 g of semolina and chickpeas
- Vegetables for couscous
- 100 g of pear compote

Dinner

- Cream of turnip curry soup
- Red cabbage salad with tofu (100 g) and cashew nuts (20 g) vinaigrette (1 tsp walnut oil)
- 100 g vanilla pudding

Sunday

Breakfast

- 150 ml fresh citrus juice
- Four wasa fibers
- 30 g of goat cheese
- Green tea

Lunch

- Avocado with lemon juice
- 100 g scallops on leeks (1 teaspoon olive oil)
- 100 g of mango carpaccio and lime

Dinner

- Velouté with coral lentils
- Fine endive tart
- One goat yogurt sprinkled with cinnamon

CHAPTER 4

SLIM DOWN BY EATING LESS MEAT

What if becoming a part-time vegetarian was the key to losing weight? Also, this new food practice is good for his body. You are told how to do it concretely.

Here are the five key principles of this diet, which allows for lightening and detoxifying by giving pride of place to foods derived from the plant kingdom.

1. Flexitarians place a premium on fresh fruits and vegetables

These fresh foods contain fiber that captures fats and toxins to eliminate them in the stool. They are also full of vitamins, minerals, and antioxidants essential to the proper functioning of the body. Finally, they fill the stomach and satiate well.

In practice:

- Vegetables are eaten at lunch and dinner, as an appetizer and as a main course, to satiety, mixing raw and cooked to enjoy maximum micronutrients without disturbing the intestines;
- Fruits containing more sugar, we are satisfied with two portions (100 to 150 g according to the fruit) per day, at breakfast, and one of the two main meals. We favor those seasonal that bring what the body needs most at this time.

2. Flexitarians ensure protein intake with cereals and pulses

Good amounts are found in legumes (chickpeas, dried beans, lentils...), cereals and seeds (whole wheat, rice, buckwheat, quinoa...) and algae.

Apart from soy and quinoa, not all of these sources provide all the amino acids (protein constituents) essential to the body: it is necessary to consume cereals and legumes during a single meal or a meal. Same day to meet his needs.

In practice:

- In the absence of meat, fish or eggs, at least one source of vegetable protein is provided;
- At one of the two meals, one consumes 150 g (cooked weight) of a mixture of leguminous + cereal (rice + lentils, chickpea + semolina ...). On the other, 50 to 100 g of soy, seaweed, or quinoa (cooked weight) are expected. We always associate vegetables.

3. Flexitarians complete with animal and vegetable eggs and dairy products

Eggs and dairy products - especially cheeses - are rich in proteins of high biological value. Vegetable juices (soy, almond, rice, oats...) and their derivatives (yogurts, creams...) also contain significant amounts. Eating each day in small quantities can supplement protein intake.

In practice:

Eggs are provided two to three times a week to make preparations (flans, pies, etc.) And natures;

And one consumes one to two dairy products per day, giving preference to those coming from small animals (goat, sheep) or vegetal versions (soy yogurt...) If cow's milk is poorly tolerated.

4. The flexitarian favors fats of vegetable origin

Unlike those contained in fatty meats, cream and butter, vegetable oils and oleaginous, polyunsaturated, are little stored by the body that uses them to renew the membranes of its cells.

In practice:

- One consumes every day 2 to 3 c. Tablespoons of various vegetable oils. For cooking, we prefer the olive, and for seasoning, we opt for rapeseed, walnut, and camelina;
- Oilseeds are also regularly included in their diet: in addition to being rich in good fatty acids, they also contain proteins! In this case, replace 1 c. Oil of the day with 20 g of almonds, walnuts, hazelnuts...

5. The flexitarian consumes meat and fish when it makes him want

Eating in excess can be potentially bad for health, especially because of the toxic substances they may contain (heavy metals in large oily fish, polycyclic aromatic hydrocarbons in processed meats...), more questions to put in the menu for lunch and dinner! But we do not hesitate if we appreciate it, especially since they also contain essential nutrients to the body (iron, zinc...).

In practice:

- Two to three times of fish and one to two times of meat a week, that's enough when you balance your plate next to it!
- We favor quality, preferring small species of fish (mackerel, sardines...) And lean morsels of meat labeled animals raised outdoors.

Vegetarian diet vs. vegan diet

Do you have trouble understanding the difference between veganism and veganism? We deliver you all the keys to see more clearly and, why not, become a follower of a diet based on fruits and vegetables.

How many vegetarians do you have around you? Three, five? And how many vegans? To help you make the difference and, why not, adopt one of these two diets, here is a little reminder of their main advantages and disadvantages.

The vegan diet

Vegan people do not eat any product or by-product of animal origin. This means that they do not eat meat, fish, milk or eggs, but not honey because bees make them. Their diet consists mainly of fruits, vegetables, cereals, nuts, and legumes.

Since animal products are the richest in protein and iron, vegans need to compensate for this lack in other ways. Lentils, soy sprouts, and beans are among the products to consume in large quantities when adopting this style of diet. Sometimes a vitamin B12 supplement is also needed. The best is to consult a doctor who tells you the best practices to follow.

Despite these restrictions that can be a bit of a pain in the daily meal organization, the vegan diet reduces levels of bad cholesterol in the blood and lowers the risk of developing cardiovascular disorders, according to a study reported by the site Medical Daily. Not to mention the impact on the environment and the protection of animals...

The vegetarian diet

The cardiovascular, certain types of cancer, and hypertension. Whether you choose to adopt or not one of these two regimes, to protect your health, that of animals or the environment, also know that "eating mainly plants has been associated with better sex life," says the site Medical Daily. A word to you...

CHAPTER 5

HOW TO GIVE UP MEAT WITHOUT GIVING UP MEAT

Meat has long had a central and very symbolic role in our dishes. Many countries with rich historical roots have long served carnivorous dishes that not only feed the population but are important cultural support. In Crete, they eat snails, sardines, and beans. In Tanzania, they eat grilled impala. Whole turkeys are carved in America to enjoy them in November. It is not that these peoples are carnivores, but that for centuries, they have appreciated the benefits of a diet that contains meat.

The indisputable fact is that meat has an extensive list of benefits for our bodies, favoring our capacity for work, growth, and exercise. Poultry, pork, veal, lamb and shellfish are essential components of our diets because they contain proteins, which are converted into energy in our body and help stimulate their daily functioning. Certain benefits are exclusive to meat consumption and cannot be substituted for vegetarian alternatives. For example, some studies have shown that red meat significantly helps neurotransmitters in our brains fight depression, anxiety, and eating disorders.

However, climate advocates begging us to replace meat with a plant-based diet to save the planet may seem to simplify the problem too much, but they are not wrong.

The slowdown in climate change is closely related to the significant decrease in our meat intake. Mass production of beef and chicken accounts for more than 18% of the world's carbon emissions. However, the decrease in our consumption of meat can be seen as a sacrifice, both culturally and nutritionally, by many populations that are not fit (either by attitude or by means) for a complete change in their lifestyle.

Framing the problem in a way that validates rather than punishes meat consumption can help us open the minds and diets of meat consumers worldwide and save the planet in the meantime. A flexitarian diet can be a good starting point. The flexitarian diet consists of a plant-based regimen but does not require the consumer to exempt the meat from their daily meals completely. Most flexitarians practice this diet by consuming many fruits, vegetables and nuts, and adding some poultry, fish, milk, and eggs in a supplementary manner.

The true beauty of the flexitarian diet is that it can fit many dishes and global delicacies without drastically changing or eliminating the fundamental aspects of the dish. For example, in Spain, traditional cuisine has many recipes with approximately 80% of vegetables and 20% of meat (such as Madrid stew), which means that the dishes themselves conform to a Flexitarian format. And, in other countries where meat is a more central component, it can be replaced with products of plant origin that do not sacrifice plate integrity.

For example, the beef necessary to make the Bolognese sauce for spaghetti, so popular in Italy, can be replaced with white beans or lentils. A Flexitarian can prepare and consume meals with any proportion of meat and vegetables depending on their region, culture, media, and personal preferences. By allowing people to decide the degree to which their diet will be based on plants, we reject the idea that one is closely vegan/vegetarian or carnivorous, and we allow any personal contribution to a more sustainable world to be recognized as such.

By changing the focus on the way we view meat consumption, recognizing its cultural heritage and nutritional benefits, we can begin to see it as a positive element rather than an enemy. In this way, we can be more open to a diet based primarily on vegetables and encourage others to do the same.

CHAPTER 6

THE FLEXITAR BURGER THAT MAKES VEGANS ANGRY

Controversy in the UK about the launch of a flexitarian burger. According to vegans, «flexitarianism» is only an advertising expedient and does not exist.

The launch of a flexitarian burger has raised many controversies in England. A fiery debate has been accessed on social media, dragging even on the national media after an intervention by a vegan activist against the latest product available in ALDI supermarkets. According to critics, "flexitarianism" does not exist and it would only be a device for omnivores to feel less guilty.

The anger of vegans against the flexitarian hamburger

What is the flexitarian burger in question? It is simply a burger launched by the Byron company that contains up to 70% beef and 30% mushrooms. It is not so much the composition that has triggered the controversy, but the choice to sell it as a flexitarian product. According to the vegan activist Laura Paterson, it would only be "squalid advertising expedient" designed only to sell more by relying on the guilt of those who eat meat "to make them feel better."

And yet, according to the activist, "The flexitarian diet does not exist, simply eat meat, or you do not eat it." Only a gimmick, therefore, designed to take hold in a growing trend and sell more hamburgers. The controversy has exploded on Facebook, turning into a real virtual counter between "vegan" and "carnivore." The story has become so huge that it ends up on the pages of several English national newspapers. Several interventions to defend flexitarianism and above all its potential as a "first step" towards a meatless diet for those who are still undecided about whether, how and when to make the transition definitively.

Flexitarianism does not exist

In England, the theme is very hot, and a greater part of the population is always choosing a vegan, vegetarian or "flexitarian" diet, reducing the consumption of meat. Like all changes in a society, it is normal for conflicts to arise. However, the question remains: does «flexitarianism» really exist or is it simply a term widely used to sell more products on the shelves? The term is still relatively new. According to Treccani, it is flexitarian: «Those who prefer to follow a vegetarian type of feeding, without giving up eating animal proteins.» This would make him, technically, an omnivore. With feelings of guilt? Maybe. Or perhaps simply with more awareness.

However, it is undeniable that there is still a certain ideological "barrier" between vegans and omnivores. Especially a certain part of omnivores. Eating meat maintains a strange aura of virility, so abandoning it is seen as an unspeakable affront to masculinity. The English have also given a name to the phenomenon: "vegetarian". Men who are afraid of vegan. At the same time, the vegan choice maintains an aura of radicalization. A choice for radical-chic. Can flexitarianism be a meeting point between the two extremes? The debate is open, hopefully, with a few virtual insults as possible.

Difference between vegetarians and vegans

The difference between vegetarians and vegans is not clear to many, although in recent years their number has increased. Let's try to make things a bit clearer.

Nowadays, you really can't help but know the difference between vegetarians and vegans. We talk about it a lot, maybe too much, almost as if following one or the other diet makes people better or worse. In reality, as always, these are merely choices. What unites vegetarians and vegans, respectively 7.3% and 1% of the Italian population (Data Eurispes 2019), is solely the fact that both have chosen to eliminate from their diet every type of animal meat, which is of land, air or water.

Here the similarities end, and two currents of thought begin, which, however similar, often find themselves in contrast. Between omnivores, vegetarians, and vegans, there is also a whole series of nuances that occasionally result in neologisms such as the Pescetarians, flexitarians and the like that also create further confusion.

What does it mean to be a vegetarian?

Following a vegetarian diet, as mentioned, means eliminating any animal food from your diet. No meat (of cow, pork, chicken, turkey) then, and no fish (including shellfish and mollusks). The term vegetarian, however, is rather vague because it indicates a category of people that it would be more appropriate to define lacto-ovo-vegetarian to differentiate them from ovo-vegetarians and lacto-vegetarians. Complicated nomenclatures are referring to those who have decided to exclude dairy and eggs from their diet, respectively. The reasons behind a vegetarian choice can be ethical (that is, dictated by love for animals) or health. In the first case, the vegetarian diet is just a transition to the vegan phase, an intermediate step towards a higher level of awareness.

What does it mean to be vegan?

When it comes to veganism, the issue becomes more complicated. Let's start by saying that those who follow a vegan diet have decided to exclude from their diet - and from their lives - as well as meat and fish, even all animal derivatives. What doesn't a vegan eat? He does not eat milk and derivatives (like cheeses); he does not eat eggs, nor does he eat honey and all those foods that in one way or another, have caused suffering to a living being. It is therefore clear that veganism is more a lifestyle than a diet based on unconditional love for living beings, from the smallest to the largest.

We have defined it as a lifestyle because being vegans often means changing most of one's daily habits, from clothing (no leather, wool, silk or fur) to leisure time (no sports like hunting or horse racing or shows that include animals like the circus or the bullfight) passing through cosmetics (choosing products not tested on animals). Seen as to fundamentalists, vegans are sometimes at the center of controversy. In reality, these are often very empathic people who, however, struggle to pass on to their peers the reasons for their choices, even if it would be nice, however, that they were never needed. Each individual should feel free to be himself, each based on his sensitivity.

CHAPTER 7

4 RULES OF THE FLEXITARIAN DIET

To fully understand how feeding a flexitarian is composed, here are the rules that those who adhere to this diet follow for their meals. The consumption of fruit (both fresh and dry) and vegetables with added meat in small doses seems to do the body very well: it lowers blood pressure, reduces cholesterol and triglycerides, and prevents cardiovascular diseases.

1. Vegetables

Organic vegetables and seasonal fruit are the focus of the diet: they are preferable to any other food, to limit the supply of baked goods and carbohydrates in general (such as bread, pasta, and rice). In this way, weight and blood sugar are kept under control. Yes, even with dried fruit, especially almonds, which have a low caloric intake but also lots of fiber and protein.

2. Whole foods, legumes, and seeds

The whole grains (barley, barley) are preferable to refined grains because richer in fiber, essential for the well-being and gut health. They are an essential part of the diet along with legumes and oilseeds. The first are beans, chickpeas, and peas (rich in vegetable proteins), the second are flax seeds, sesame seeds, pumpkin seeds. All these seeds contain omega three and omega six which help to lower bad cholesterol and raise the values of the good one.

3. Animal proteins and derivatives

In the flexitarian diet, there are, however, animal proteins, unlike the vegetarian diet; their presence serves the muscles to keep themselves toned. Even if in very limited quantities, therefore, meat, fish, eggs, and dairy products are allowed. In exceptional cases, you can introduce sausages, canned meats, and smoked meats.

4. Rediscovery of regional recipes

The regional recipes of the Mediterranean diet have an excellent balance of nutrients, especially proteins. For this reason, the flexitarian diet aims at the rediscovery of those traditional dishes that combine health and taste: from pappa al Pomodoro originating in Tuscany to orecchiette with Apulian turnip greens.

CHAPTER 8

FLEXITARIAN RECIPES

Are you looking to reduce your meat and fish consumption towards a different way of life that is more respectful of your environment? Are you looking for vegetables and seasonal products, and want to cultivate dietary diversity, by cooking more plants? Welcome to our section dedicated to flexitarian! Here you will find all our easy and fast recipes to help you choose a semi-vegetarian diet, allowing you to eat a good piece of meat or a fish fillet now and then!

Puree of sun vegetables with basil and olive oil

   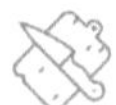

Dish for four people

Preparation: 10 minutes

Cooking time: 30 minutes

Level: Easy

Ingredients

- 400 g eggplants
- Two bouillon cubes KUB DUO® Vegetables & Herbs MAGGI market
- 400 g of zucchini
- 400 g potatoes
- One tablespoon of liquid cream
- 1/2 tablespoon of olive oil
- Five chopped basil leaves

Preparation

1. Peel the potatoes and cut into cubes. Wash zucchini and eggplant and cut into cubes as well.

2. In a Dutch oven or casserole, bring a liter of water to the boil, add the broth cubes, vegetables and cook for about 30 minutes.

3. Drain the vegetables and pass them to the mill to obtain a puree. Mix, add the liquid cream, olive oil, and chopped basil. Sip immediately.

Vegetable moussaka

   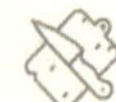

| Dish for eight people | Preparation: 15 minutes | Cooking time: 55 minutes | Level: Easy |

Ingredients

- Two zucchini
- Three eggplants
- One bouillon cube KUB DUO® Vegetables & Herbs MAGGI market
- 100 g of feta
- One onion
- One can of 400 g of tomato crushed (240g net weight drained)
- One briquette of Béchamel Sauce MAGGI (350ml)
- Two tablespoons chopped basil
- Two tablespoons breadcrumbs
- One clove of garlic
- Six tablespoons coarse salt

Preparation

1. Cut the aubergines into 5mm thick slices and let them disgorge in a colander 30 minutes after salting them generously. Rinse with cold water and wipe dry.
2. Chop the onion and garlic. Cut the zucchini and feta cheese into small cubes.
3. Brown the aubergines in a hot pan with a tablespoon of oil, reserving them on paper towels. Throughout cooking, add a little water to make them melt.
4. Preheat the oven to 180 ° C (Th.6), in the same pan fry the onion, garlic, and zucchini for about 5 minutes, add the crumbled broth cube, tomatoes, and basil. Cover and let simmer for 10 minutes.
5. In a gratin dish, arrange a layer of eggplant, then a layer of zucchini preparation, alternate the layers and finish with aubergines. Top with bechamel sauce, feta, and sprinkle with breadcrumbs.
6. Cook 40 minutes, the top should be browned.

Peppers stuffed with cereals

   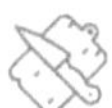

Dish for eight people

Preparation: 15 minutes

Cooking time: 25 minutes

Level: Easy

Ingredients

- One red pepper
- One green pepper
- Two yellow peppers
- 250 g of bulgur
- Two balls of mozzarella
- 150 g tomato pulp
- One stick Maggi Mixes Parfaits Italian
- One onion

Preparation

1. Cut the mozzarella into small cubes. Cut the peppers in half, keeping the tail, seed them. Make them precook hollow face up 5 minutes under the grill of the oven.

2. Cook the bulgur for 10 minutes in boiling water. Chop the onion and brown for 5 minutes in the pan with a spoonful of oil.

3. Mix the bulgur, the onion, the stick, and the dice of tomatoes, the dice of mozzarella (keep some dice to put on it). Garnish the peppers, add a little mozzarella. Spend another 5 minutes under the oven grill.

Tartines with small vegetables

   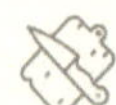

| Dish for eight people | Preparation: 30 minutes | Cooking time: 10 minutes | Level: Easy |

Ingredients

- Two capsules of BROTH CORD MAGGI® Vegetables
- Four slices of country bread
- 200 g of beans
- 100 g of peas
- 80 g of fresh, natural goat cheese
- Eight medium tomatoes
- One onion
- One tablespoon of oil

Preparation

1. Peel and chop the onion. Incise the tomatoes and cook for 3 minutes in a pan of boiling water. Peel and seed them. Cut them into small dice.

2. In a frying pan, fry the onion with the oil for 5 minutes, add 100 ml of water and let reduce, add the tomatoes and a heart of broth, prolong cooking for 2 minutes — Reserve in the fridge for 1 hour.

3. In a saucepan of boiling water, cook the beans and peas for 10 minutes. Drain them, add the remaining broth heart, and the fresh goat cheese: mix and mix.

4. Serve these preparations separately on slices of toasted country bread cut in half.

Homemade taboule

   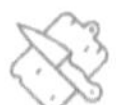

Dish for four people | Preparation: 15 minutes | Cooking time: 5 minutes | Level: Easy

Ingredients

- 200 g of medium semolina
- One capsule of BROTH CORD MAGGI® Vegetables
- Three beautiful tomatoes
- 1/2 cucumber
- 25 g raisins
- Ten mint leaves
- Two lemons
- Six small white onions
- Four tablespoons of olive oil
- One pinch of pepper

Preparation

1. Swell the grapes in a little hot water. Book 10 minutes.

2. In a saucepan, boil 1/4 liter of water and two tablespoons of olive oil and pour the semolina out of the heat. Stir, cover, and let swell for 5 minutes.

3. Add the Bouillon Heart Capsule and mix until melted and refrigerated.

4. Wash, seed tomatoes, and half cucumber and cut into cubes. Chop the onions and mint leaves.

5. Mix all the ingredients with the semolina by adding the juice of the two lemons and the rest of the olive oil. Serve your recipe taboule very fresh.

Rice with mushrooms and leek fondue

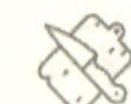

| Dish for three people | Preparation: 10 minutes | Cooking time: 15 minutes | Level: Easy |

Ingredients

- 200 g of Paris mushrooms
- One capsule of BROTH CORTE MAGGI® Garlic & Parsley
- One leek
- 120 g cooked white rice
- One shallot
- One tablespoon of sunflower oil

Preparation

1. Wash the vegetables. Cut the mushrooms into thin slices, slice the leek, and the shallot.

2. In a frying pan with the hot oil, brown the mushrooms, leek, shallot, and cook for about 5 minutes on high heat.

3. Cook the rice. Drain it and add the broth heart and the vegetables, mix.

Chickpea and vegetable salad

   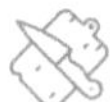

Dish for four people | Preparation: 15 minutes | Cooking time: 10 minutes | Level: Easy

Ingredients

- 200 g chickpeas
- Four carrots
- Two zucchini
- One stick Maggi Mixes Parfaits Oriental
- One onion
- One eggplant
- Two tablespoons of olive oil
- 50 g raisins

Preparation

1. Cut the vegetables into cubes of 2 cm. Slice the onion.

2. Brown, the onion for 5 minutes with the oil, add the zucchini, eggplant, grapes, and carrots and cook for 12 minutes covered with 200 ml of water.

3. Add the stick, the chickpeas, mix and place in the refrigerator for 1 hour.

Moroccan pepper salad

   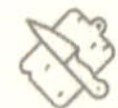

| Dish for four people | Preparation: 10 minutes | Cooking time: 30 minutes | Level: Easy |

Ingredients

- Two red peppers
- One stick Maggi Mixes Parfaits Oriental
- Two yellow peppers
- One green pepper
- One tablespoon of olive oil
- One tablespoon lemon juice

Preparation

1. Cut peppers in half. Make them black on a baking sheet under the grill 30 minutes. Place them 10 minutes in a freezer bag and remove the skin. Cut them into strips. Mix the stick, the olive oil, and the lemon juice. Pour on it.

2. Refrigerate for 1 hour.

Gratin of pears and turnips — Bakery style

Dish for four people | Preparation: 10 minutes | Cooking time: 60 minutes | Level: Easy

Ingredients

- 450 g turnips
- Two cubes of bouillon KUB OR MAGGI
- 450 g pear
- 350 g carrots
- ½ liter of water
- Two tablespoons of olive oil
- One pinch of pepper

Preparation

1. Preheat your oven Th 8 (240 °C)
2. Peel turnips, peas and carrots, and slice. Mix them.
3. Dilute the two tablets of Kub Gold in the water according to the instructions.
4. Oil the gratin dish with the brush and pour the vegetables. Pepper. Add Kub Gold.
5. Place on the rack of your oven and cook for about 1 hour.
6. Serve immediately.

Moroccan and bulgur salad

Dish for four people

Preparation: 15 minutes

Cooking time: 10 minutes

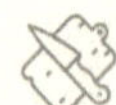

Level: Easy

Ingredients

- Five oranges
- 100 g of bulgur
- One stick of Maggi Mixes Parfaits Oriental
- 20 mint leaves
- 20 leaves of parsley
- Two tablespoons of olive oil

Preparation

1. Peel the oranges and cut them in thin slices. Keep the juice.

2. Finely chop mint and parsley. Cook the bulgur in boiling water for 10 minutes, let cool.

3. Arrange the oranges on four plates, add the bulgur and the herbs. Mix the stick in the juice and olive oil. Pour on it. Refrigerate for 1 hour.

Cakes with Auvergne Blue and nuts

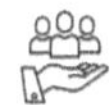

Dish for six people

Preparation: 10 minutes

Cooking time: 20 minutes

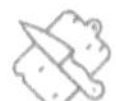

Level: Very Easy

Ingredients

- 100 g of Auvergne Blue
- 350 ml of semi-skimmed UHT milk
- Three eggs
- 50 g crushed walnuts
- One packet of MOUSLINE Nature Puree
- One sachet of baking powder
- One tablespoonful of flour

Preparation

1. Preheat your thermostat oven 8 (240 ° C) in the traditional model. In a bowl, mix 350 ml milk, the bag of puree, the eggs, the flour, and the yeast.

2. Add diced blue and crushed nuts.

3. Pour in a 6-piece muffin pan and bake 20 to 25 minutes. Wait 10 minutes before unmolding

Terrine of grilled vegetables

 Dish for six people

 Preparation: 10 minutes

 Cooking time: 45 minutes

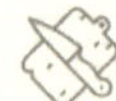 Level: Medium

Ingredients

- One beautiful zucchini
- One tablespoon Aroma MAGGI
- 200 ml unsweetened condensed milk
- One eggplant
- Three eggs
- Three tablespoons flour
- Two tablespoons chopped basil
- Two tablespoons of olive oil
- One pinch of salt
- One pinch of pepper

Preparation

1. Preheat your oven Th. 7/8 (220 ° C).

2. Wash and slice the vegetables. In a large frying pan with hot oil, fry the zucchini and eggplant over high heat for about 2 minutes. Add the Aroma and continue cooking over medium heat for about 5 minutes. Stop cooking and add basil — salt, pepper, and mix.

3. Mix half of the vegetables with the basil and two tablespoons of water. In a bowl, whisk the eggs with the milk and flour. Add the mixed vegetables.

4. Butter a cake tin. Line the bottom of half of the grilled vegetables. Pour half of the mix. Make a layer of grilled vegetables, then pour the rest of the preparation.

5. Bake in your oven for about 35 minutes.

Small carrot and zucchini flans

   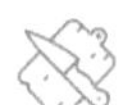

Dish for five people | Preparation: 10 minutes | Cooking time: 25 minutes | Level: Very Easy

Ingredients

- One small zucchini
- One onion
- One capsule of BROTH CORD MAGGI® Vegetables
- One carrot
- 300 ml of semi-skimmed UHT milk
- Two eggs
- One tablespoon flour
- One knob of melted butter for the ramekins
- One pinch of pepper

Preparation

1. Preheat your oven Th.7 / 8 (220 ° C). Peel the carrot. Wash and grate the vegetables. Peel and chop the onion.

2. In a nonstick frying pan, fry the vegetables and onion for 2 minutes over medium-low heat, add the heart of broth capsule, pepper, and mix.

3. In a salad bowl, mix the eggs, the flour, the milk, add the cooked vegetables.

4. Butter 5 ramekins, pour the mixture and cook for about 25 minutes.

Ratatouille Nicoise

   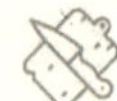

| Dish for four people | Preparation: 10 minutes | Cooking time: 20 minutes | Level: Easy |

Ingredients

- One zucchini
- 2 MAGGI® BOUILLON® HEART CORD capsules Mediterranean Vegetables
- One tomato
- One small eggplant
- One red pepper small
- One small green pepper
- Two tablespoons of olive oil
- One pinch of pepper

Preparation

1. Wash the vegetables. Peel the eggplant, peel the peppers. Cut tomato in four, diced peppers and other sliced vegetables.

2. In a skillet, heat the oil. When it is hot but not steaming, add Bouillon heart capsules and vegetables. Stir — pepper and cook over medium heat for 10 minutes while mixing.

3. When the mixture begins to melt, continue cooking over low heat until vegetables are cooked, about 15 minutes, stirring occasionally.

4. Cover if necessary at the end of cooking.

Sweet and sour vegetables

Dish for four people

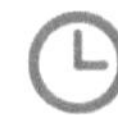

Preparation: 15 minutes

Cooking time: 20 minutes

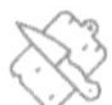

Level: Medium

Ingredients

- Four slices of pineapple in syrup
- Two tablespoons of Arome MAGGI
- Three zucchini
- Two carrots
- One onion
- Four tablespoons tomato sauce
- Four tablespoons of wine vinegar
- Four tablespoons of sugar
- Two tablespoons of oil
- One ginger knife tip

Preparation

1. Peel the carrots and cut them into cubes, as well as the pineapple slices and zucchini. Peel and slice the onion.

2. In a saucepan containing the hot oil, cook the carrots for about 5 minutes. Add zucchini and pineapple cubes and onions and cook for another 10 minutes.

3. Add the vinegar, the sugar, the aroma, the tomato sauce, the ginger then prolong the cooking of 5 minutes. Serve.

Lemon eggplant caviar

   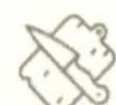

Dish for two people | Preparation: 15 minutes | Cooking time: 10 minutes | Level: Easy

Ingredients

- Two eggplants
- One onion
- One stick of Maggi Mixtures Parfaits Italian
- The zest of 1 half lemon
- Two tablespoons of olive oil

Preparation

1. Chop the onion. Peel and dice eggplant.

2. In a frying pan, brown the onions with the oil for 5 minutes. Add the eggplants and continue cooking for 10 minutes. Add the lemon zest and the stick — Mix 1 minute.

Smoked duck breast and crushed potato

   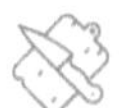

Dish for four people | Preparation: 10 minutes | Cooking time: 10 minutes | Level: Easy

Ingredients

- 100 g smoked duck breasts
- Two bags of mashed potato flavored mashed potatoes
- 250 g of forest mushrooms
- 300 ml of semi-skimmed UHT milk
- One tablespoon chopped parsley
- 400 ml of water

Preparation

1. Brown the chopped mushrooms for 5 minutes in a pan with the chopped garlic and half the parsley. Prepare the puree according to the instructions for use with half the parsley.

2. Add the pieces of duck breasts to the hot mashed potatoes.

3. Serve the duck breast in a circle and add the mushrooms.

Cocotte of spring vegetables

   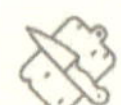

Dish for four people | Preparation: 15 minutes | Cooking time: 30 minutes | Level: Easy

Ingredients

- Four new carrots
- 1 KUB Bouillon KUB DUO® Vegetables & Herbs MAGGI market
- Four new potatoes
- Four small turnips
- One red onion
- 500 g fresh green beans or 100 g frozen
- One clove of garlic
- One tablespoon brown sugar
- 10 g of butter

Preparation

1. Peel all the vegetables. Cut carrots and potatoes into thick slices, turnips, and red onion into wedges.

2. Cook the beans in a saucepan of boiling salted water for 5 minutes, then drain and set aside.

3. Place the carrots in a pan, add the broth, crushed garlic clove, butter. Cover with water and cook for 10 minutes undercover. Add the other vegetables and continue cooking for 15 minutes covered. Add the beans and continue cooking for 2 minutes.

4. Using a skimmer, remove the vegetables. Arrange them on the plates and keep warm. Let the broth reduce with the brown sugar and coat the vegetables. Serve.

Bruschetta with artichoke

   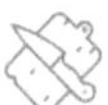

Dish for four people | Preparation: 15 minutes | Cooking time: 20 minutes | Level: Easy

Ingredients

- Three artichokes
- Eight slices of bread
- One stick Maggi Mixes Parfaits Italian
- Two tablespoons of olive oil
- Two tomatoes
- One clove of garlic
- Two tablespoons lemon juice

Preparation

1. Cook the artichokes 15 minutes in the pressure cooker with 800 ml of water. Seed and cut the tomatoes into small cubes.

2. Remove the leaves and hay. Keep the leaves and cut the heart into small dice.

3. Mix the artichoke cubes, the stick, the oil, and the lemon juice. Add tomatoes and refrigerate for 1 hour.

4. Toast the bread and rub the garlic on it. Cover each toast with artichoke and serve immediately!

Sautéed forest mushrooms, small potatoes, green beans

Dish for four people

Preparation: 10 minutes

Cooking time: 22 minutes

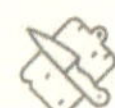

Level: Easy

Ingredients

- 400 g of a mixture of frozen or fresh forest mushrooms (cepes, boletus...)
- 1 MAGGI® Garlic & Parsley Broth Capsule®
- 200 g small potatoes
- 300 g green beans
- One tablespoon of olive oil

Preparation

1. To make your pan-fried forest mushrooms, small potatoes, and green beans, start by baking the green beans, wash the vegetables.

2. In a saucepan with boiling salted water, pre-bean green beans, and potatoes for about 10 minutes.

3. In a frying pan containing the hot oil, fry the mushrooms for about 2 minutes, then add the potatoes and green beans, cook over medium heat for about 7 minutes.

4. Add the broth heart capsule and continue cooking over low heat for about 3 minutes.

Crispy triangles with vegetables

 **Dish for eight people**

 **Preparation:** 10 minutes

 **Cooking time:** 15 minutes

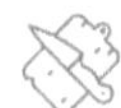 **Level: Easy**

Ingredients

- 6 Sheets of Brick HERTA
- One capsule of BROTH CORTE MAGGI® Garlic & Parsley
- One eggplant
- One zucchini
- Two beautiful carrots
- 10 g of butter
- Two tablespoons of olive oil

Preparation

1. Preheat the oven to Th.7 / 8 (220 ° C). Peel and cut the carrots into sticks. Wash and cut the eggplant and zucchini in small cubes.

2. In a pan containing the oil, fry the vegetables for 5 minutes over medium heat. Add the broth heart capsule and mix until melted.

3. Cut the pastry sheets in half and place them rounded down.

4. Place vegetables on the top left and folded the corner to form a triangle. Fold again twice. Brush with melted butter and place on the baking tray covered with parchment paper — Cook for about 10 minutes.

Wheat with pineapple, pepper and coconut milk

 Dish for four people

 Preparation: 10 minutes

 Cooking time: 20 minutes

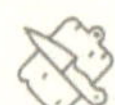 Level: Easy

Ingredients

- 800 ml of water
- Three sticks of Bouillon KUB OR MAGGI
- 300 g pre-cooked wheat
- One box of 165 ml of coconut milk
- One tin of 140 g pineapple in sliced syrup
- One red pepper
- One untreated lime

Preparation

1. Slice the pepper.
2. Drain the pineapple and cut it into pieces.
3. Wash and chop the lime zest, then squeeze the juice.
4. Carry the water and the sticks of Kub Or to boiling and add the wheat. Cook for about 20 minutes, until the water is completely absorbed.
5. Five minutes before the end of cooking, add the pineapple pieces, the juice, the zest of the lime, and the coconut milk.
6. Finish cooking on low heat, pour into a serving dish, and enjoy immediately.

Vegetarian burger with lentils

   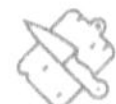

Dish for three people | Preparation: 15 minutes | Cooking time: 6 minutes | Level: Easy

Ingredients

- Three plain burgers
- One bag of Mousline puree Curry Lentils & Potatoes
- One egg
- 100 g of cottage cheese 20% of natural fat
- Two tomatoes
- One half red onion
- 50 g of corn salad
- 200 ml of semi-skimmed UHT milk
- 100 ml of water
- Three cheeseburgers

Preparation

1. Preheat your Th.8 oven (240 ° C) in rotating heat.

2. Mix the milk, 100 ml of water, the bag of puree, and the egg. Separate into 3. Make three flat steaks between two sheets of parchment paper. Remove the top sheet — Bake for 6 minutes in the oven.

3. Cut the tomatoes into slices. Slice the onion. In each burger, add the cottage cheese, tomatoes, a steak, cheese, and bake for 3 minutes in the oven. Add onion and lamb's lettuce. Close and serve immediately!

Puree tricolor with cream

   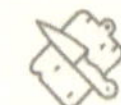

| Dish for four people | Preparation: 30 minutes | Cooking time: 20 minutes | Level: Very Easy |

Ingredients

- 500 g of vitelotte potatoes
- One packet of MOUSLINE Nature Puree
- 2 Kub Bouillon KUB Poultry MAGGI
- 500 g carrots
- 300 + 250 + 100 ml of semi-skimmed UHT milk
- 15 g of butter
- Two tablespoons fresh cream 30% fat

Preparation

1. Prepare the Mousline puree according to the instructions for use with 250 ml of milk and 500 ml of water, add the butter and mix.

2. Peel and cut the carrots into slices, pour into a pan with 100 ml milk, and half the stock — Cook undercover and on a low heat for 20 minutes.

3. At the same time, peel and cut the vitelotte potatoes into slices and cook them in 300 ml milk with the remaining bouillon cube — Cook under cover and on a low heat for 20 minutes.

4. Add the carrot puree to the blender and crush the vitelotte potato with a fork, add a spoonful of cream in each mashed potato. Serve this puree in verrines or for children, have fun, and draw a character on the plate.

Crumble with southern vegetables and parmesan

 Dish for four people

 Preparation: 15 minutes

 Cooking time: 12 minutes

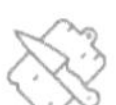 Level: Easy

Ingredients

- 1/2 yellow pepper
- 1/2 red pepper
- One capsule of BROTH HEART® MAGGI® Mediterranean Vegetables
- 1/2 onion
- One zucchini
- 30 g of butter
- Three rusks
- 15 g of flour
- One tablespoon shaved parmesan grated
- One teaspoon of oil

Preparation

1. For a crumble with southern vegetables and parmesan, preheat your oven Th.7 / 8 220 ° C. Chop the onion and cut the vegetables into small cubes. In a frying pan, fry with the oil for 8 minutes, add the broth heart capsule, and cook for 3 minutes. Divide into four ramekins.

2. Mix butter, finely crumbled crackers, flour, and parmesan cheese. Sprinkle over the crumble — Bake in your oven for 12 minutes.

Veggie burger with lentils and quinoa

   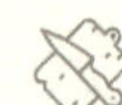

| Dish for four people | Preparation: 00 minutes | Cooking time: 20 minutes | Level: Easy |

Ingredients

- 300 g cooked lentils
- 100 g of quinoa
- One stick of Bouillon KUB OR MAGGI
- Two onions stem
- Four buns
- Two eggs
- Eight big pickles
- 100 g of cottage cheese 20% of natural fat
- Ten sprigs of chives
- One teaspoon of curry

Preparation

1. Slice onions and brown for 5 minutes in the pan. Cut four gherkins into slices and chop the rest. Add the cottage cheese and chives.

2. Mix lentils, cooked quinoa, eggs, onion, and crumbled broth and curry. Form 4 steaks and fry for 3 minutes on each side.

3. Garnish each burger with cottage cheese and steak.

Vitamin plate: Chinese cabbage and roasted pumpkin

 Dish for four people

 Preparation: 15 minutes

 Cooking time: 25 minutes

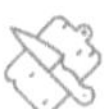 Level: Medium

Ingredients

- 400 g of pumpkin
- 280 g of blond quinoa
- 1/2 Chinese cabbage
- Two cubes of Bouillon KUB OR Reduced Salt MAGGI
- Two tablespoons of olive oil
- 1 liter 500 of water
- 30 g of hazelnuts

Preparation

1. For the pumpkin: Preheat, the oven to 200 ° C., Cut the pumpkin into eight slices with the skin. Place on a baking sheet. Sprinkle with olive oil and crumble a cube of Kub Gold Salt Reduces Maggi® on it.

2. Bake for 15 to 20 minutes. The pumpkin must be melting. For the quinoa: prepare a broth with a Kub Gold Reduced Salt Maggi® cube and 1 liter of water. Pour the olive oil into a saucepan and fry the quinoa. Cover with hot broth and bring to a boil. Lower the heat, cover with a lid and simmer for 10 minutes.

3. Drain, keep some cooking water, and put the quinoa back in the pan with the lid to keep warm.

4. For Chinese cabbage: remove large leaves on the outside. Slice the cabbage finely. Heat the olive oil in a pan and add the sliced cabbage. Brown. Salt and pepper. Add a little water, cover, and braise for about 10 minutes. Cabbage must be "al dente."

5. For training: Crush the hazelnuts. Make a quinoa sauce in a bowl or soup dish. Place two slices of roasted pumpkin and a little braised cabbage. Decorate with crushed hazelnuts. Sprinkle with quinoa juice.

Vegetable curry

(Vegetables) Curry always works! This delicious and simple dish from Southeast Asian cuisine is unmatched in terms of diversity. By adding a variety of spices and ingredients, you can quickly prepare your favorite curry. In our variant, we completely abstain from meat. Broccoli, zucchini, and peppers are our main ingredients. The addition of fresh pineapple finally makes our curry flexitastic. How that works, we show you here.

Ingredients (4 servings)

- One medium-sized broccoli
- 2-3 peppers
- One medium-sized zucchini
- One small fresh pineapple (alternative: pineapple from the tin)
- spring onions
- 100 ml vegetable broth
- 500 ml of coconut milk
- 1 tbsp curry powder
- 1 tsp turmeric
- One teaspoon green curry paste
- One teaspoon yellow curry paste
- One teaspoon paprika powder
- chili flakes
- Salt pepper
- One tablespoon soy oil (alternative: olive oil or coconut oil)

Preparation

1st step: preparing vegetables

1. Wash the vegetables thoroughly. Divide the broccoli into small florets, peel the stalk with a peeler and then finely dice. Core the peppers and cut into 2 cm pieces. First, slice the zucchini and then dice. Cut the spring onions in about 1 cm wide rolls. Set everything aside.

2nd step: preparing curry

1. For the vegetarian vegetable curry, heat the oil in a large saucepan at medium temperature. First, put the peppers and zucchini in it. Then add broccoli and spring onions and fry them together with the turmeric. Season with salt and pepper and then deglaze with the vegetable broth and simmer briefly.

2. Now add the coconut milk, reduce the heat, and gradually add all the remaining spices.

3. The whole now simmers under a closed lid for about 20 min.

3rd step: complete curry

1. The sharpness in the curry can be combined very well with the sweet pineapple. While the curry is simmering, cut the pineapple into pieces and add to the curry for the last 5 minutes of cooking time.

2. Put the prepared vegetable curry in a small bowl and sprinkle with chili flakes. For this vegetarian vegetable, curry fits best Basmati rice.

3. We wish you good luck with cooking and a good appetite.

Falafel burger with sweet potatoes

The falafel comes from the Arabian cuisine and consists mainly of chickpeas. Normally, the falafel is served in the form of small balls. From this delicious chickpea food, you can easily create flat patties that are perfect for our veggie burger. Our vegetarian falafel burger tastes best with oven-fresh sweet potato fries.

Ingredients

- Two bread rolls of your choice
- 200 g of chickpeas flour
- fresh parsley
- cumin
- Two shallots
- One tomato
- iceberg lettuce
- One red onion
- One ripe avocado
- 200 g of natural yogurt
- 1 tbsp mustard
- paprika
- Salt pepper
- Four tablespoons olive oil

Preparation

1st step: prepare falafel

1. Boil 150 ml of water in a kettle.
2. Peel the shallots and cut into fine cubes. Wash the parsley (amount as you like) and finely chop. In a large bowl, mix the chickpea flour, shallots, and parsley — season with a pinch of salt and two teaspoons of cumin. Slowly add the boiling water slowly and slowly until a sticky mass is formed. Attention: It should not have a too liquid consistency, otherwise rework with a little bit of chickpea flour.
3. Set the falafel dough on its side and let it rest for 15 minutes.

2nd step: preparing burgers

1. For our veggie burger, we use two different sauces - yogurt and avocado.
2. For the yogurt sauce, mix the yogurt with the mustard and season with salt, pepper, and rose paprika. If you want, you can also add some lime juice.
3. For the avocado cream, remove the shell of the avocado and crush the fruit with a fork to a creamy consistency — season with salt, pepper, and, if desired, with a little garlic powder.
4. For the burger, topping peel, the red onion and cut into rings, wash the tomato and slice it and wash some salad, shake dry, and set aside.

3rd step: prepare falafel patties

1. For the falafel patties, heat plenty of olive oil in a medium-sized pan.
2. In the meantime, add 1 tbsp of olive oil to the falafel dough and knead with moistened hands. From the mass, then form two flat patties.
3. Then sauté the patties from each side for about 5 minutes in the pan until they have a golden-brown crust.

4th step: prepare falafel burger

1. Halve the rolls. Then place the burger in the following order: yogurt sauce, lettuce, tomato, falafel pattie, avocado cream, onion rings.
2. As a side dish, homemade sweet potato will taste the best fries from the oven.

Stuffed kohlrabi schnitzel with vegetable fries

Stuffed schnitzel with a difference! It does not always have to be meat - the proof is in this simple and tasty dish. Kohlrabi schnitzel stuffed with cheese and wrapped in a crunchy breading. Also, light and healthy vegetable fries of carrots and beetroot. Test it fast, and you will see: you'll love it!

Ingredients (2 servings)

- One large kohlrabi
- 5-6 carrots
- One medium-sized beetroot
- Four slices of Emmentaler
- 200 g of natural yogurt
- Breadcrumbs as needed
- One medium egg
- Salt, pepper from the mill
- 1 tbsp olive oil
- Three tablespoons of butter lard or heat-resistant oil (eg, thistle oil)

Preparation

1st step: preparing vegetable fries

1. For the vegetables, peel carrots and beetroot with a peeler and then cut into pegs. Tip: Use kitchen gloves for the beetroot so that your hands are not completely red afterward;-).
2. Mix the vegetables with chips in a bowl with the olive oil, season with salt and pepper, and spread on a baking sheet lined with baking paper.
3. Preheat the oven to 180 degrees.

2nd step: Prepare kohlrabi schnitzels

1. For the kohlrabi schnitzel, fill half of a pot with water and bring to the boil on the stove - add two tablespoons of salt.
2. Meanwhile, peel the kohlrabi with a peeler and remove each end with a knife. Now divide into equal slices (it is best to choose an even number, as two slices are required for one schnitzel).
3. Put the kohlrabi slices in the boiling water and cook for about 8-10 minutes over medium heat.
4. Now the oven should be preheated, and the vegetable fries can be put on the middle rail in the oven (about 25 min).

Step 3: Finish kohlrabi schnitzel

1. After the cooking time, drain the kohlrabi slices and allow them to cool briefly.
2. Meanwhile, whisk the egg on a plate and spread the breading on another plate. Also, provide the Emmentaler in slices. Now season the cooled kohlrabi slices with salt and pepper. Cover each half with the cheese and then put the other half over it, pass it through the egg, and finally cover with the breading. Repeat this procedure for each chip.
3. In a pan, heat the clarified butter and fry the kohlrabi schnitzel in it from each side for about 3-4 minutes at a moderate temperature.
4. Put the kohlrabi schnitzel on a plate and serve with the vegetables.

Broccoli buffer with a fresh herb quark dip

Broccoli instead of potatoes today! Varied and colorful should be a healthy kitchen - for this reason, it is green today. A healthy and delicious alternative to potato pancakes is these spicy broccoli buffers. Served with a dip of quark and fresh herbs, this dish can be seen.

Ingredients (2 servings)

- 300 g of broccoli
- One onion
- One clove of garlic
- 5 tbsp olive oil
- 30 g almond flour
- One tomato
- Salt pepper
- some chives
- 150 g of low-fat quark
- Two tablespoons natural yogurt
- One teaspoon freshly pressed lime juice
- Two eggs
- 40 g of grated Parmesan

Preparation

Step 1: Broccoli mixture

1. Preheat the oven to 180 degrees upper and lower heat. Rinse the broccoli carefully underwater and divide it into small florets. Peel the stalk and finely dice. Peel the onion and garlic, finely dice and mix with the broccoli and one tablespoon of olive oil. Season with salt and pepper. Place the mixture on a baking tray, cover with a baking paper and cook in the preheated oven on the middle rack for approx. 12 min.

Step 2: Quark dip

1. Remove the broccoli mixture from the oven, place it in a bowl and allow it to cool briefly. Wash the tomato, remove the stem stems, remove seeds and then finely chop. Rinse chives under water and cut into fine rolls. Mix the quark, yogurt and lime juice, season with salt, pepper, and various herbs. Add the diced tomatoes and the chives to the dip and set aside.

Step 3: Completing the broccoli buffers

1. Add the eggs, parmesan, and almond flour to the broccoli mixture and let it swell for 2 minutes. Heat 2 tablespoons of oil in a pan. Add 2-3 tbsp of the batter to the pan, fry each side for 1-2 minutes until golden brown on medium heat. Remove the fried buffers from the pan and drain briefly on a kitchen crepe. Serve buffer with dip.

Vegetable curry

(Vegetables) Curry always works! This delicious and simple dish from Southeast Asian cuisine is unmatched in terms of diversity. By adding a variety of spices and ingredients, you can quickly prepare your favorite curry. In our variant, we completely abstain from meat. Broccoli, zucchini, and peppers are our main ingredients. The addition of fresh pineapple finally makes our curry flexitastic. How that works, we show you here.

Ingredients (4 servings)

- One medium-sized broccoli
- 2-3 peppers
- One medium-sized zucchini
- One small fresh pineapple (alternative: pineapple from the tin)
- spring onions
- 100 ml vegetable broth
- 500 ml of coconut milk
- 1 tbsp curry powder
- 1 tsp turmeric
- One teaspoon green curry paste
- One teaspoon yellow curry paste
- One teaspoon paprika powder
- chili flakes
- Salt pepper
- One tablespoon soy oil (alternative: olive oil or coconut oil)

Preparation

1st step: preparing vegetables

1. Wash the vegetables thoroughly. Divide the broccoli into small florets, peel the stalk with a peeler and then finely dice. Core the peppers and cut into 2 cm pieces. First, slice the zucchini and then dice. Cut the spring onions in about 1 cm wide rolls. Set everything aside.

2nd step: preparing curry

1. For the vegetarian vegetable curry, heat the oil in a large saucepan at medium temperature. First, put the peppers and zucchini in it. Then add broccoli and spring onions and fry them together with the turmeric. Season with salt and pepper and then deglaze with the vegetable broth and simmer briefly.
2. Now add the coconut milk, reduce the heat, and gradually add all the remaining spices.
3. The whole now simmers under a closed lid for about 20 min.

3rd step: complete curry

1. The sharpness in the curry can be combined very well with the sweet pineapple. While the curry is simmering, cut the pineapple into pieces and add to the curry for the last 5 minutes of cooking time.
2. Put the prepared vegetable curry in a small bowl and sprinkle with chili flakes. For this vegetarian vegetable, curry fits best Basmati rice.
3. We wish you good luck with cooking and a good appetite.

9 781710 131789